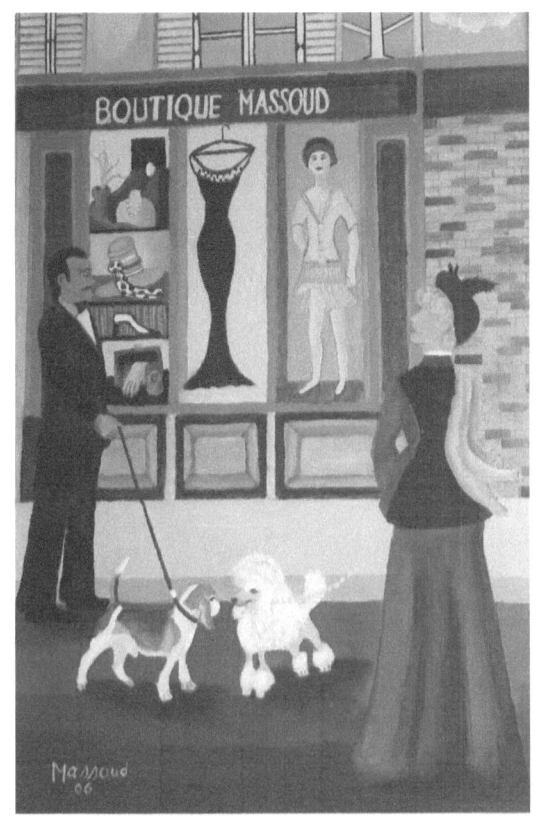

OVER EIGHTIES

Massoud Eghrari M.D. F.A.C.S

authorHOUSE®

AuthorHouse™
1663 Liberty Drive
Bloomington, IN 47403
www.authorhouse.com
Phone: 1 (800) 839-8640

Published by AuthorHouse 04/30/2018

ISBN: 978-1-5462-4085-3 (sc)
ISBN: 978-1-5462-4086-0 (e)

Library of Congress Control Number: 2018905290

CONTENTS

ACKNOWLEDGEMENTS

As this is a work of non-fiction, in order to protect privacy, the identity of some individuals and places have been disguised.

The author wishes particularly to thank his wife, Tayebeh (Manijeh) for her assistance and encouragement. Also thanks his lunch group for listening to his reading every Wednesday.

Also special thanks to Kathy Hemmat for her patience in typing the manuscript.

WHY THIS BOOK?

My daughter Jackie was on vacation at my house. I saw her reading a book and smiling. I asked, "What is the book's name and what is it all about?" She said, "It's called *Over Fifty*. It is about all the trials and tribulations of people over fifty years of age."

Then like a bolt of lightning hitting me, I said to myself, "Why not write a book about the over eighties?" I had never heard of such a book. I went to the internet to see if anyone had written such a book. But I didn't find any.

Today the group of over eighties is growing in number every day thanks to modern medicine. I believe they will be interested to read this book and see their common trials and tribulations. As well as enjoying the common moments of happiness and laughter.

Thus, the book of *Over Eighties* was born.

AGING GRACEFULLY

Aging gracefully is a myth. How can anybody age gracefully? God has given the geriatric people very little tools to accomplish this.

How can they do it with no hair on the scalp, no functioning teeth in the mouth, and no good memory left in the brain? They have pain in the arms, legs and back; indigestion and diarrhea and constipation. How can they age gracefully?

This is a propaganda that old people have been saying to each other for centuries to keep their morale up and be able to continue on.

Aging gracefully depends on your money. If you have a lot of it, you can live more comfortably. You can buy better food and have better medical care.

Recently I was watching a program on television. They were interviewing an old man of ninety years of age who previously was CEO of Vanguard Mutual Fund. He definitely has aged gracefully because of his money. Twenty years ago at the age of seventy, he had a heart transplant to keep him in good shape. If he did not have money this would have been impossible. It is all about money.

It also depends in whose eyes one is aging gracefully. Is it by the eyes of a stranger or by the person himself?

One aspect that most agree with, is that aging gracefully is a lot easier when one has money but also when one is able to maintain a state of good health!

ALL IS IN THE ANKLES

For the past eight years, I have been studying the feet and ankles of the people walking on the sidewalk of Gulf Shore Blvd. Every morning when I walk there I try to understand why people walk so differently from each other and I try to guess their age according to their walk.

I came to the conclusion that all is in the movement of the ankle and not in the foot. If the ankle is stiff, one walks like Japanese women with a tight kimono dress. This person is old and most likely has severe arthritis. If the ankle is supple and one walks with fully bended ankle he is middle-aged and sportive. If the ankle is loose and the person jumps when he walks, he is a teenager.

According to my observation, the age of a person can be determined by the movement of the ankles. I can guess his age, not by looking at his face and counting the wrinkles or by the color of his hair but rather by the movement of his ankles.

All is in the ankles!

CELEBRATION

Last night I went to the celebration of the one year anniversary of the passing of my friend. His wife had organized this meeting and she had invited a group of his close friends to talk about his life and their memory of him. The guests were mostly over eighties and his contemporaries.

While I was sitting there I turned to my wife and said, "Take a good look at all these people, because in five years from now more than fifty percent of them will not be here." This was a sad statement.

But when I looked around and reexamined the audience I saw three groups. The first group was standing at the side of their grave, the second group were very close to the grave, and the third group, the younger folk, were standing far away. I knew most of them. I knew their medical history and I knew scientifically that the demise of the first and second groups were imminent. But in the case of the third group death could happen without any warning.

In either case, there was no guarantee about who goes first. Then I remembered when I was taking my walk before Hurricane Irma I could see some very old trees that have only a few green leaves on their branches and there were some younger ones with a lot of green leaves. However, after the hurricane, some of these old trees survived while some of the younger ones were pulled out of the ground and died. Then I came to the conclusion that it does not matter how much knowledge or statistics we have, we still cannot predict the moment of death.

COMMUNICATION

I don't like communicating with email, text, twitter or snapshot. I am from the old school. I like to pick up the telephone and talk and discuss. I feel unsatisfied using electronic devices.

However, the younger generation, don't want to talk, they don't want to move their tongues. I am afraid that if they continue that way, their tongues will atrophy and even possibly fall out of their mouths!

I am not familiar with computers. I would call myself "illiterate computer savy". I type with one finger. I look for each word intensely and I am so happy when I find it. It takes me about one hour to type one page.

I use the computer to read my email and look at the stock market. Occasionally I get to a website of some establishment for specific information, then by mistake, I touch something on the keyboard and I lose the page. And I can't get it back! It is very frustrating to be a dinosaur in this time of electronics.

Yesterday, I received a letter from the Department of Education of the state of New York to renew my license to practice medicine. The letter said that this year we purchased a fancy computer that can renew your license very easily and you can also pay your dues.

But there was no place for an old fogey like me who does not know how to navigate computer science. I did not know how an illiterate like me could accomplish my renewal. I called the Department of Education. After listening to their music, finally, a gentleman answered. I explained to him my dilemma. He was surprised that a doctor of medicine did not know computer science. He reluctantly said, "We will send you a paper application and you can send it back by mail."

This license can only be renewed for two years. I don't know two years from now - when I will be two years older - if they will allow me to renew it by paper. But I doubt I will become proficient in computer science by then.

COSTCO

Yesterday it was a rainy day, I could not go to the beach, nor to the pool. I said to my wife today is the right day to go to Costco. When we arrived, the parking lot was crowded. I guess everyone also had the same idea. In the rain I ran to the entrance. As usual the old lady at the door wanted to see my membership card. I put my hand in my pocket and pulled out my wallet. It had many cards shoved into it. One could not see any of them clearly. I just half-opened the wallet and showed it to her. Of course, she could not see Costco's card but she made believe that she saw it and let me in.

When I was inside I saw two elderly disabled persons, each riding a motorized shopping cart. They were playing and following each other, like kids with the Bumper Cars.

First I went to look at jewelry cases. I said to myself, "Why anybody with brains would come to Costco to buy jewelry?" But after awhile I saw they had 18 karat gold and 3 karat with SI1 and F rating diamond.

I continued my journey by pushing the cart. This was Saturday about noon and many old ladies were advertising food and giving free samples. If one wanted to eat a complete lunch, he could start sampling food, from chicken nuggets to fish to cheese to bread. Then he could continue to have dessert with cookies and fudge. Then top it off with coffee and finally get a mouthwash, before leaving.

I saw again the motorized disabled couple. On the tray in front of them they had all kinds of food that they had gathered during their promenade.

As I continued my rounds, I saw people going inside a huge refrigerator, picking up delicate fruit and vegetables. Then running out, like as if a beast was chasing them.

Finally, I get to the cashier. I put all of my stuff on the counter and a young Spanish looking girl checked them out very quickly. I had no time to verify if she was doing it correctly. Then she said $257.00 dollars. I said $257.00 is too much it must be a mistake. We are only two people and there is no way we can eat that much. But she showed me the screen and I realized that I had bought a large amount of food because I thought it was cheap. I really did not need that much. I was sure we would never be able to eat all of it. A good portion of it will end up in our garbage bag.

Soon after leaving the cashier, in the restaurant, I saw the same people, who had eaten their way through Costco sampling all kinds of food. Now they were sitting and devouring hot dogs, pizza and ice cream.

As I was going out I saw many items advertised for sale. Among them was a coffin with bronze handles and shiny wood. I came to the conclusion that if one eats his way through Costco he would surely need a coffin sooner or later.

When I exited the store, another old lady checked me out by looking into the shopping cart. I could not believe that realistically she could see everything in this crowded basket by a blink of her eyes. She made believe that everything was okay and she let me out.

When I got to the parking lot I felt like I had a good day and said to myself in Costco not only can you buy anything on earth but also you can eat free, and be entertained by watching people.

DEPRESSION

Depression is common among the over eighties. It has been estimated that 1.6 percent of people age sixty-five and older have depression. I have seen it in several of my friends. They get disappointed with life due to problems with their children and grandchildren. They get disappointed with their investments and especially in their health. As a result, they give up and go into hibernation.

Depression increases with age: 2.8 percent at the ages of 18 to 24, 4.8 percent at ages 46 to 64 and the percent is even more for the over eighties.

How to overcome depression? 1) Fight with oneself to become an optimist. The optimist lives five years longer than the counterpart the pessimist. 2) Have a partner or friend to talk over the problems of life. 3) Have good nutrition. It is like putting high-test gasoline in the car, it works better. 4) Stimulate the brain by learning new things like a foreign language, music and solving puzzles.

The alternative is not any better. People with depression develop heart attacks four times more than regular people.

DIET

This morning my wife asked me, "What would you like for breakfast?" Without any hesitation I said, "Two eggs over easy." She replied, "You had two eggs yesterday and how about your cholesterol?" I said, "At this stage of my life I don't believe two eggs would make any difference in my health.

This reminded me of one of my friends in Long Island, who was about ninety years old. One day when we had a meeting in our house he took me aside and said, "I have to ask you a question." Then he pulled a long file from his packet. This was a report of all his recent lab works. He said "Look at my cholesterol. It is elevated. What should I do?" I looked at him with a smile. I said, "Enjoy your life and don't worry about your cholesterol." It does not matter how old you are. You just want to follow a healthy diet.

For over eighties, our goal should be "The preparation for a good death." We should eat all natural and organic foods. We should exercise every day. We should keep our minds active. We want all lab work to be perfect; all CT scans normal. Because we do not want to be sick when we die!!

If we are not in good health, we will linger around. Society would treat us with the latest treatment, latest surgery, latest drugs. Only to extend our lives in misery. We don't want to die with oxygen in our noses, a feeding tube in our stomachs. Or leg amputated due to uncontrolled diabetes.

Our ultimate goal should be to have an autopsy that shows that we were in excellent health before the day we died! Therefore follow a healthy diet.

DOCTOR'S OFFICE

I don't go to the doctor every day or even every other week. I go maybe once in every six months! I go to the doctor like a baby goes to a well-baby clinic. But when I see a doctor I expect a lot. This is entirely my fault. I compare their service with the service I rendered to my patients. But alas, everything has changed and managed care has ruined it.

After searching for an internist for some time a friend recommended a doctor who newly opened her office. I called her for an appointment. The secretary said, "Not so fast. First, we are going to send you a four-page questionnaire about the state of your health. When we receive it back, the doctor is going to review it and see if she wants to accept you as a patient."

When I received the application, not only did I answer all the questions from my childhood up to the present, I also gave full information regarding all members of my family. Then I waited and waited. Finally, they called me and gave me an appointment.

I had no idea who the doctor would be and how old she would be. All I knew was that she was a woman.

On the appointed day I went to her office. The nurse

practitioner greeted me and questioned me more and took my vital signs. While I was waiting for the doctor I was imagining the size and look of her. I was hoping for a good-looking woman.

Finally, the door opened and a very skinny, short girl entered. She was dressed in blue jeans and a blouse. Her black hair was pulled back behind her ears. She looked like a teenager in high school.

She was pushing a portable computer through the door with difficulty and needed my help. She said, "I know everything about you. I have read your dossier carefully and then she examined me from head to toe and declared me in good health. This was the first time that somebody had touched me.

In general, the doctors in Naples follow a non-touch technique. This means they look only at the computer while talking to you and never touch you.

The whole experience was not satisfactory. I need a doctor who is fatter, taller and older - not a shrimp. But I was thankful that finally, I have found a doctor who accepted me!

DOG LOVERS

Gulf Shore Blvd. in Naples, Florida has a lot of high-rise building apartments. Their inhabitants are mostly older retired people and many of them own dogs. These dogs are not ordinary, small dogs. They are pure-bred.

In the morning, all owners walk their dogs and converse and compare the different medications their dogs need. It is like a "Dog Convention". But I feel very bad for the dogs. They are stuck with old people and mostly old ladies. These dogs deserve to be owned by a young ten to fourteen-year-old kid who will play with them and wrestle with them.

But unfortunately, they have to live with these geriatric people. They want the dog because they are lonely and in need of a loving companion. It is good for them but not for the dog.

I see the poor dog on the beach. They want to run but due to the poor condition of their owner they cannot do it.

Sorry dogs!

DRIVING

Most over eighties drive in Naples, FL. They usually own the latest model of a famous car factory such as Mercedes, Lexus, Infinity and sometimes Rolls Royce. The drivers put the top down enjoying the sun and the wind while their few white hairs are blowing in the breeze.

Their driving is not the best in the world and if they would take the driving exam again they would surely flunk! They don't know where they are going and in the middle of the road without warning they slow down and sometimes stop while they are looking for the number of the building or the sign of a store.

This reminds me of the story of an old couple who moved to Naples from New York City. The wife asked the husband to go to the drugstore to get her special prescription. The drugstore was about eight miles away from their house and he had to take the highway to get there.

When the man left his wife she was watching television. Suddenly she saw "Breaking News!" The reporter said, "There is a car with New York license plates driving the wrong way on the highway." The woman immediately called her husband and asked, "How are you doing?" He answered, "In this neck of the woods, there is an amazing phenomenon. The people are all driving on the wrong side of the road. I am the only one going the correct way!"

Now one sees the caliber of these drivers.
God save us all!

EXERCISE

It is the opinion of experts that the elderly should exercise every day. According to a research paper published in the Journal of Geriatrics, the residents of nursing homes who walk every day, even short distances, live longer than the ones who remain lying down or sitting.

With this argument in hand, lots of elderly in Naples, Florida walk every day on the sidewalks of Gulf shore Blvd. or on the beach. These people before coming to Florida never exercised. Now that they are in warm weather, they wear shorts and a tee-shirt, and they show their very white skin to the world. They want to exercise to the highest level. But there are lots of dangers.

Their equilibrium is not good. Falling is a major problem. I have often seen drops of blood on the sidewalk and I imagine they have come from a poor elderly person who wants to become a champion by fast walking.

I do not want the reader to think that I am critical of the elderly. I am one of them. But in order to not show my age, I walk every day about three miles and swim about 30 minutes. I recently read in the Journal of Neurology that if you exercise too much, it will kill you too. Excessive activity will put too much pressure on your arteries. Moderation! Moderation!

EXPIRED MERCHANDISE

When I go to the CVS Pharmacy to pick up a prescription the pharmacist puts a label on my bottle that states my name, the name of the medicine, and finally the expiration date. This expiration date means that the drug most likely is obsolete after a certain date and in some cases may be dangerous.

In the same manner, when I go to the supermarket, I see that most merchandise has a shelf life. When the manager sees that the expiration date has passed, he throws all expired products into the garbage.

I said to myself, "Everything has an expiration date, why not human beings?" Maybe the date should be stamped on our foreheads. This would be particularly useful when you meet someone for the first time. You would look immediately at his forehead and you see how much time he has left. If he only has one month, you may not want to become friends with him!

I am writing all this preamble, because tonight watching the news, Brian Williams reported that life expectancy now depends upon where you live. Then he said, "If you are a man and live in Fairfax, Virginia, the average life expectancy is 81 years". I said to myself, "Did I hear him right? Did he say 81?"

Then I said, "I must be expired merchandise because soon I will be 87".

That night I dreamed I was in Costco, where there was a concentration of elderly people. I saw all the people had a yellow tag on their clothes saying EXPIRED! I looked at myself and I did not have a yellow tag. I wondered, "Why not?"

I came to the conclusion that probably my Creator has appointed a stupid inspector to check out and dispose of all expired humans. When he looked at his list he misread my year of birth! Instead of 1930, he read 1950. Therefore, he passed me by.

At this point, I said to myself, "You should not call anybody to correct the mistake. Definitely, keep quiet. If the inspector finds out his error, he may come back and you will be in trouble." Then I woke up I was happy that at least for a while, I was 20 years younger!

FAT IS GOOD

An old person should not be skinny! He or she needs some amount of fat for reserves. If he gets sick, he will lose weight and this is the time he will need to use his reserve. This is like having money in a savings account for a rainy day.

Fat accumulates in the omentum which is like an apron inside the belly that covers the intestines. Also fat accumulates in the buttocks and breasts. Nature calls on this reserve when needed, especially when the person cannot eat or when he is traumatized for some reason.

One should forget the propaganda about being skinny. Your heart and lungs can handle a certain amount of weight gain. I know this is contrary to the advice of cardiologists but this is a lesson from my past experience.

Now that we are on the subject of fat, I have to tell you about my experience at a restaurant. Recently I was at a fancy restaurant. The menu was extensive and the food was good. I wondered who the chef was and what he looked like. In my opinion, if the chef is fat, the food is good, because he tastes the food all day and he likes eating. If the chef is skinny obviously he does not like the food and his product will not be good.

With this theory in mind, I asked the waitress to see the chef. When he came out, indeed he was fat and I was happy that my theory was proven to be correct. Fat is good!

FLYING WITH EAGLES

In Persian, we have an expression that says, "Pigeons fly with pigeons and eagles fly with eagles." On our trip in the United Kingdom, we were flying with eagles: bald eagles, white eagles, disabled eagles, female eagles and male eagles.

Forty of us riding in a luxury bus and traveling from the south to the north. We were all above seventy and had a lot in common – the same type of disposition and almost the same type of complaints. Our bladders were in the same condition and the bus would stop every two hours for a bathroom break.

We had no pigeon with us to complain and pick on us and be impatient. We were all very accommodating. No one runs and walks fast. No one could do it anyway. It was reassuring that we were all in the same boat.

Most of the eagles were very educated and knowledgeable. They had already traveled around the world and they knew what to do and what to eat. On this trip, everything was good except the food. British food has a bad reputation to the point that in France if they want to let you know that the food is tasteless they call it - à *l'anglaise*. Like the boiled potato – they call it *Patato à l'Anglaise*.

At the end of this trip, all the eagles survived and were brought to Edinburgh Airport to fly home.

FREE LUNCH

Every week I receive several invitations to come to a seminar with lunch in a nice restaurant. I have never been interested to respond but when I received a professionally printed card in a bright red envelope I said to myself, "They are after me so I better respond!"

I called the place and a man answered. He had a gruff voice that sounded like the Godfather. He was in a hurry and all he wanted was my name and address.

In the invitation, they were talking about building a condominium in Bonita Springs with a lot of fancy accoutrements. I thought it would be nice to go and see what they are offering and do a comparative price study with the price of my apartment and be reassured that in the current real estate market I had not paid too much.

When I arrived there on time at 10:30 a.m., I was surprised to see that the restaurant was already overcrowded. The time of the lecture was 11 a.m. This gave me a hint that these people were all elderly retirees who didn't have breakfast and were hoping for an early lunch!

The man who spoke was about 50 years old with white hair and a good-sized belly. His voice was warm and pleasant.

He explained to us that all the apartments for sale were for the lifetime of the occupant. When the owner dies, 92 percent of the entrance fee would be refundable to his heirs. He went on to say that the occupant's would be provided with food, entertainment and, medical treatment. There would even be a section for Alzheimer patients.

When he said the word, "Alzheimer", I felt uncomfortable and frightened. I didn't expect this kind of talk. My condition was not that bad. Then I looked around to evaluate the audience. They were all very old and frail. Many of them had visible deformities and some were carrying their portable tanks of oxygen.

The salesman continued to talk and tried very hard to frighten this poor, old folks by telling them, "If you suddenly developed a heart attack or stroke, and you are not in our condominium complex with the latest medical devices, no one would know about you. Like Elvis Presley, your body would be discovered the next day.

After this intimidating talk I started fidgeting in my seat and did not want to be there. I felt sorry for the frightened seniors who in my clinical judgment were ready to go to their grave and on their way this man wanted to collect all their money.

The salesman was such a convincing speaker, that even I felt that if I did not buy an apartment from him, I would regret it the rest of my life.

He was in the middle of his talk when I felt that I could not take it anymore. I looked around for some way out. Fortunately, I saw the sign of the restroom. I tiptoed out and left the room. When I returned, I was happy to see a plate of classical Tilapia fish was at my place. When I started eating, I looked again at the audience and I saw all these disabled, old people had come alive, devouring their food, like this was their last supper.

Then I said to myself, "Who said there is no free lunch in this world? There is one at the Bonefish Grill, and these old folks are here for it!"

FRIENDSHIP

Long lasting friendships generally start in elementary school or high school or even at college. But for over eighties it is rare to start it at this age. People are more standoffish and even suspicious. This situation does not apply to our small group of over eighties.

Our group varies from three to eight but the basic number who lives most of the time in Naples is four. We go to lunch every Wednesday, to talk, to laugh and enjoy two hours feeling free to speak our minds.

The subject varies from the situation in our building or the beautification of Gulf Shore Blvd. to sometimes national politics. Because we are old, all together we make a very interesting museum of illness. But rarely do we talk about our miseries. We do talk plenty about medical care in this town and in the nation.

Our group is diverse in every way. Our Dean is a retired pediatrician who has tried his hand at politics and almost became a state senator. He also was an entrepreneur and an accomplished musician. As an American Italian he enjoys good wine and a good cup of espresso.

The next in line is a bon vivant, retired podiatrist. He is

always happy and in a good humor. He collects jokes and makes us laugh. Although he is an Italian American I have never seen him drink wine or enjoy espresso.

The next is a retired undertaker. He is always very quiet and does not speak very much. But when he does we all listen to his pearls of wisdom.

The last is me. I am the newcomer to the group, an American Iranian from a third world country. A retired breast surgeon who paints and writes and plays music. I don't drink alcohol but do drink water without ice.

Though we are all from different parts of the United States: Rhode Island, Upstate New York, Michigan and Long Island, New York, we never get angry at each other, even when the topic of conversation is politics.

It has been proven that friendship, as well as laughing, extends the life. I am honored to be part of this group and to spend my Wednesdays with them.

GENERATION GAP

This is not a myth. It is real. The new generation does not want to play with us old folks. The first time I saw this phenomenon was when I was invited to a party at my daughter's home. Most of the guests were around their mid-forties. After greeting me and talking about some superficial subject I was totally ignored. They did not want to play with me.

They were deep in discussion about their own common problems and their solutions. At no time did they ask my opinion and if they had I don't think they would have accepted it. I felt rejected and lonely. I said to myself, "This is the law of nature." Then I remembered the following story about when I was in my fifties:

I was part of a group of people my own age who once a month would get together in someone's home to discuss subjects from Us States Department book regarding the world's problems.

In one of these meetings, the mother of our host was present. She was visiting her daughter for a week. She was a lady over eighty with white hair and a raspy voice. She was dressed like a woman of forty. She was well-educated with a PhD degree.

Each time she would open her mouth to say something and participate in the discussion, the guests would not pay any attention to her. I also was wondering why she was meddling in our conversation. Her ideas were old-fashioned and not for today.

As you see, what goes around, comes around. Indeed there is a *"Generation Gap."*

THE GERIATRIC REVOLT

They came to this cruise from all over the world. No one forced them to be here. But why did they come? Because they did not want to be considered old and forgotten. But deep down they knew they were not young. In reality they were revolting against the world and their society. They wanted to retake their legitimate place in society and be just as they were many years ago.

Tonight they wanted to be treated like teenagers. They were on the dance floor. They were happy, they were loud, and some were drunk. This was something pathetic, yet exciting to watch.

in one corner I could see a husband and wife dancing and holding each other like two lovers who just met. But when I looked closer I saw that their large bellies prevented them from any intimate contact.

On the other side of the floor I saw an old man jitterbugging with a young girl. But unfortunately, his arthritis has affected him so much that he couldn't do what he wanted.

In another corner I saw an old lady sitting in a wheelchair

suddenly get up and ask her husband to help her get to the center of the dance floor.

As the night progressed the old people did not want to leave. Their revolt was successful. When the music stopped they were back again to the reality of life!

GERIATRICS

I hate the word *"Geriatric."* It makes me sad and even nervous. In my imagination, a geriatric person is an old man who has a few sparse, white hairs on the top of his head. His face is haggard with big grooves on his pale cheeks. His neck has a mass of extra skin hanging down, like a turkey's neck. His chest is like a barrel and his belly protrudes. His buttocks are almost non-existent and his legs are skinny and hairless like two pieces of wood. In truth, he is standing at the edge of his grave and ready to jump in.

But society does not want him to die. Everyone wants to keep him healthy and alive. For this reason, they have created a Department of Geriatrics in hospitals and there is a Geriatric Physician on duty. In my opinion, this is an age discrimination to segregate the old people in one place. This should be against the law.

When you talk to the members of this geriatric tribe they think they know everything and they argue that their life experience has made them special chosen people. In spite of all this, I don't want to belong to this "Tribe".

Yesterday I had an appointment to see my cardiologist for a routine yearly check-up. He did an echocardiogram, asked me a lot of questions regarding my health and examined me. When all was done he said, "You are a healthy octogenarian!" To him, it was a compliment, but to me, it was not. This was the first time I heard the word, octogenarian attributed to me. I was depressed all day. I did not want to be called "octogenarian". In my mind, I thought I was "*Sexagenarian!*"

But alas, I am an octogenarian. The clock cannot be turned back. It doesn't matter what I think, in truth, I am one of these geriatric people and I should be proud of it.

I am trying.

GOOD DEATH

My friend Jay from Long Island called. He was one of my referring physicians and a member of our discussion group. We had a nice conversation talking about current affairs and reminiscing about the past. When he was going to hang up he said, I wish you a happy day and a good death." When he hung up I started to think, I felt that this was not an insult instead it was a good wish.

I don't want to have a bad death. I don't want to be disabled. I don't want to be bedridden and I don't want to be fed by a tube. In order to have a good death, I have to be in good shape. For this reason, I walk three miles every day and I swim 30 minutes. I am interested in my health like putting money aside in a savings account. This way when death comes I would not be a heart cripple. I would not be an amputee due to diabetes. I would not be paralyzed. I would be a perfect statue of health.

This is controversial but when I think about it, it is true. I have seen some of my patients lingering around in a miserable condition for years; they are having a bad death.

Wishing someone a good death is a good wish!

HARD OF HEARING

The majority of over eighties are hard of hearing but they don't admit to it and blame it on the T.V. and as remedy they turn the volume up. This will continue until the day that they go for a hearing test.

Twenty years ago my wife was complaining that the television's sound was too high and I must be hard of hearing. With her insistence, I made an appointment to see an Ear, Nose and Throat Specialist. Before going I said, "Maybe you should come with me and have your ears checked too."

We both arrived at the doctor's office. He and his technician tested our hearing. Then we were brought to his office to listen to his verdict and each one of us receive our sentence.

He was smiling when he opened the door. He said, "I can't believe my findings." Then he looked at me and said, "You have no problem with hearing. But your wife needs hearing aids." She was shocked and of course did not accept the verdict and sentence.

Since that day I have seen three Audiologists for evaluation and each one told me that I don't need hearing aids. But the problem is that sometimes I don't get what I am hearing.

My feeling is that all is not due to the problems of the internal ear. It maybe is the brain. The distance between the ear and the brain gets longer and longer when we get older. It will take more time for the brain to decipher and analyze the sound he receive. Therefore we don't always understand quickly the words. It is like delayed transmission when reporters on TV talk to each other from two different corners of the world.

But with all these theories in mind, I had to go back to the Audiologist for another check for the fourth time. Yesterday I saw the Specialist MD with a Fellowship in ear disease. After extensive evaluation and testing, he said, "You may benefit from wearing a hearing aid."

My feeling is that if you shop long enough, eventually someone will sell you a hearing aid!

P.S. I tried hearing aids - there was no improvement and I gave them up!

HEALTH

Recently I was reading the March issue of AARP magazine when I noticed the article about "Health". It was saying that when you get to the age of eighty, in most cases, you don't have to have a colonoscopy, mammogram, P.S.A. test and Pap smear. I am sure this is because it is not cost-effective. The feeling of authority was that you have lived your life and you will die of something eventually. If we spend all this money on the old folks there will not be much left for the treatment of the young and middle-aged.

But the thing that society does not know is that these over eighties have a lot of power. They elect the president, governors, senators, etc.; and they have a lot of money.

There is still hope for this group. They can get rejuvenated and back in circulation. They can get plastic surgery, they can get blood or plasma transfusions from the blood of young people. They can physically be in contact with young people to feel younger.

Many people with a lot of money are working in this direction. They want to be young again. Such as Larry Ellison – co-founder of Oracle, Larry Page, CEO of Google, and Peter Thiel, co-founder of Pay Pal. They believe that man can live to the age of one hundred and eighty.

You see: There is still a lot of hope for
all these "Over Eighties"!

INDEPENDENCE

For the over eighties independence is very important. I don't want people to think I need help because I am old! Recently I went to Macy's department store to buy a shirt. When I got to the cashier I decided to use cash rather than a credit card. Since I was not used to paying with cash, I was fumbling with my money to get the exact change. The cashier, a nice looking woman, perhaps felt that I was too old and didn't know how to calculate. She started getting in my wallet to help. I didn't like it at all! I told her that I am alert and capable of doing my business and didn't need her help.

Also, I like to drive my own car. I am very capable to do it. I have never had any accident and have never gotten a ticket. But sometimes my wife suggests that she should be the driver rather than me. I don't like it. I think that if I don't drive I will forget how to. Then I will become disabled.

Last night we were at the Baha'i Feast. The hostess had prepared the readings and was handing them out to each guest. When she got to me she said, "If you think this reading is too long you can read just half of it and pass it to the next person." I thought she felt I was too old and wouldn't be able to finish it. Then the lady next to me said, your reading is very long and mine is short. We can exchange." I did not like that idea. I am old, but I am still capable. Maybe I am getting paranoid.

I hope I won't ever need any physical help and I can remain independent!

INVITATION TO LUNCH

Yesterday, late in the afternoon, I went to my mailbox to pick up all my mail from Friday, Saturday, and Monday. I usually don't pick up my mail on Friday and Saturday because if there is any disagreeable letter, I cannot contact anybody and I will have the *heebie jeebies* all weekend.

At the mailbox, I found a lot of correspondence. Among them was a brightly colored yellow envelope, similar to the color of Persian lemon. I didn't want to wait until I got upstairs to my apartment to open it so I hurriedly opened it with my fingers in the hallway in front of the mailboxes.

The card inside was professionally printed. On top of it, I could see in capital letters: "Invitation to Lunch." The restaurant was the Capital Grille in Naples, Florida. The host had given me a choice of two days – Tuesday, April 25, and Thursday, April 27. On both days the time was 11:30 AM. There was a telephone number to call to make a reservation but I could not see who was inviting me.

At this time I was anticipating eating one of their juicy steaks with the customary shrubbery around it. I was almost tasting it. Then I looked inside of the envelope to see if I could find any other information. I found a green colored paper tucked inside. I pulled it out and started staring at it.

It was from an organization I had never heard of before by the name of the "American Society of Cremation". I was surprised. How did they know that my demise was soon forthcoming? Who gave them my name? How do they know how old I am?

I continued to read further. There was a list of their services with the cost. I said to myself, "Why are there different prices from one thousand to several thousand? Is it not the same flame? Do they use a special color in the fire? Do they sprinkle gold on the fire? Do they use an expensive perfume?

I was so disgusted with this invitation that I didn't want it to contaminate the rest of my letters. I simply dropped it in the garbage in front of the mailboxes!

LONGEVITY

Recently I read an article about longevity and what factors may improve it. The article said, "You don't gain many years because you eat well, live in a fresh air region, exercise or are skinny. Only two factors are most important. One is having a very close friend that you can rely on and is your confidante to discuss any problems, no matter what. The second one, which is at the top of the list, and makes your life longer, is the number of people who you come in contact with every day. The more contacts the better.

When I read that I said to myself, "I should start contacting all the people I know. The closest person was my wife, next was my doorman. Then I contacted all of my friends and talked to them.

When I finished, I decided to calculate to see how many hours all this would increase my life. After working with my calculator I came to the conclusion that I would gain five hours of life each day. Then I multiplied five hours by 365 days and it came to be 1,825 hours which would translate to seventy-seven days. I deducted fifty per-cent or 38 days for not contacting the people at night. The final grand total was thirty-nine days.

This meant that every year I would have potentially added one month to my life. In five years I will have gained five months. I questioned myself if it is really worth it to go through all this trouble and spend that much time and effort to gain only five months? Then I said, "Of course it is! Because in all this contact one receives love and affection which are important factors for a happy life."

So go out of your way and talk to all
of your friends every day!

MAINTENANCE

When I was working, I would start at 7 a.m. and operate all morning. In the afternoon, I had office hours where I would see my pre and post-op patients. In the evening I had dinner with my family. Occasionally at night, I would get calls from Emergency rooms to go there to see a patient and possibly perform an operation. In summary, I was busy full-time taking care of others.

Now that I am retired and living in Florida, my entire time is devoted to taking care of myself. What I mean to say is taking care of my body. This has become a full-time job!

I am up at 6 a.m. Then at 7:30 a.m. I go for a walk. One hour later I return and it's time for breakfast. Next, I watch a program on TV. At 9:30 a.m. the stock market opens and I want to see what is happening in that department. At 11 o'clock I have to make my telephone calls: doctor's offices for appointments, pharmacy for renewal of my prescriptions, call to Comcast to fight with them regarding my internet or television bill.

Then it's time for lunch. Afterwards, I take a one hour nap. This is a must! When I wake up I go swimming. And after that, it's time for dinner. By this time I am tired, I need some relaxation. I sit on the couch in front of the TV and watch some stupid program while I doze on and off. Then it is time to go to the real bed for the night.

In summary, I am involved on a full-time basis to take care of myself. I have realized I am not rendering any service to anybody else. Looking back, I don't know how I worked full-time and took care of myself at the same time.

I have a friend who has no interest in life other than taking care of his body. He spends a great amount of time to detoxify himself by taking laxatives and enemas three times a week. For hours, he juices all kinds of fruits and vegetables. He goes a long distance to a special store to buy organic food. He never goes to any parties or sees any movies. His reading is all about information that tells him how to live a healthy and long life. I just don't know if it's all worth it. I hope one day he doesn't get hit by a truck. Then all of his past efforts would have been for nothing!

My conclusion is that we old people of Florida are like the working horses that are sent out to pastures to spend the rest of their life in leisure. We should enjoy life and not be worried that we don't perform now as when we did when we were young. We have been there and we have done that!

MANNERS

The over eighties believe that no one has good manners anymore in this world. If they do have it is much less than when they were young. They think that the new generation, under the pretext of freedom and a state of relaxation, have destroyed good manners. What is even worse, they are not teaching them to their children.

Good manners may be outmoded but they are the niceties of life. Young people don't dress well when they go to theaters, restaurants, churches or when they are traveling by plane.

Recently I had dinner at Capital Grill in Naples. The restaurant is known for its chicness and its service. My wife and I were sitting close to the window and celebrating her birthday. The hostess brought two couples to the table next to us. I looked at the two gentlemen in the group. I noticed they were wearing shorts. They were not dress shorts like Bermuda shorts, they were the shorts of bathing suits. I told my wife, "I can't believe that the maître d allows them to be seated in this restaurant." She said, "They have money, why not?"

Then I remembered many years ago when I went to the Plaza Hotel in New York City for an afternoon tea. They were known for their high tea and an orchestra that played classical music. I was dressed properly in a suit and tie and my wife was wearing a long dress. When the maître d greeted us he said, "Sorry, sir you can't come in." I was surprised as to why. He said you are wearing sneakers and this is not permitted. This was then. But now people have forgotten all these good manners.

Part of having good manners is treatment of women by men such as running in front and opening the door or not sitting in the car until she is securely in her seat. But because of equality of women and men, women have decided that they don't want all of this gallantry.

I hope that good manners will come back and the new generation will teach their children of these niceties of life.

MENTAL SLOWNESS

The over eighties are not physically and mentally quick. The word takes a long time traveling from the ear to the brain to be analyzed, even though the distance between the ear and brain is quite short. It is said that the majority of these old folks are hard of hearing. It may be so, but the problem is not only hearing it is also understanding and interpreting by the brain.

Forgetfulness is the first stage of Alzheimer's in many cases. I have many friends that when we get together they repeat their life story over and over again. To them, it is the first time. Yesterday I was sending some bank statements from my computer to my printer. With a great difficulty, I accomplished it. Then I decided to write down each step so that the next time it will be easier to do. When I started, I found that I had already forgotten all the steps!

I got very depressed and angry at myself. But what is a person to do? Is there any treatment? I have seen a lot of advertisements for different medications to improve the memory but none have been approved by the F.D.A.

My memory is very important to me. I have a good

reputation to remember the past. It is a gift that I can remember the details of things that happened many years ago. Now I don't want to lose this gift. I am praying to remain alert and sharp to the last minutes of my life.

MORRIS

Two weeks ago I suddenly developed pain in my shoulders, neck, and hip. The pain became severe at night to the point that I could not sleep. For the first two days, as most patients do, I treated myself with anti-inflammatory and analgesic drugs, but there was no relief. Then due to my wife's insistence, I called my Rheumatologist's office- knowing that it would be difficult to get an appointment on the same day– I told the secretary that my pain was so severe that for the past two nights I could not get any sleep and now I am exhausted.

She listened to me and put me on hold. After five minutes of listening to country music, she came back and said, "I found a spot for you at 11 a.m. today."

When I saw the doctor I explained to him my symptoms. He said, "I think you have Rheumatoid Arthritis and the only thing I can do is prescribe cortisone." I replied, "I don't like all the side effects. Isn't there some other medicine?" He put his reading glasses on and looked through my file. I told him that five years ago I had the same symptoms and then you gave me an anti-malaria drug that cured my symptoms. He said, "You have a good memory. You are right!" . Then he told me that this medicine takes two to three weeks to take effect.

"I believe you should take the cortisone, but before taking it, I want you to have several blood tests."

I left the office somewhat depressed. The reason for this was that after five years my symptoms had recurred. That night without taking any cortisone I slept well and the next morning I had no pain. I was very happy. I said to myself, "This is a miracle! I should celebrate and go to Nordstrom's and buy several new shirts." When I arrived at the store I said to myself, "be careful don't improve your appearance so much that you become like Morris."

Morris was a bachelor about 50 years of age. He was chubby, his hair was matted together and had not seen a barber for a long time. His teeth were crooked and yellow. His clothes were old and shabby. The only thing he knew how to do was work, work, and work. One day when he was in his store he had a heart attack. He was taken to the hospital in critical condition. When he was in the I.C.U. he talked to God. He said, "I promise if I recover I will completely change myself and become a different man!"

After weeks in the hospital, he survived and was sent home. Then he started to see the barber for his hair, and the dentist for his crooked teeth. He bought all new clothes. He was so much changed that women were very attracted to him and he eventually got married.

One day he said to his wife, "I want to go to a picnic at the top of a mountain. When they got there suddenly the weather changed and there was thunder and lightning. The lightning struck Morris and killed him and he went to Heaven. When he came before God he asked God, "Why did you not take me when I was ugly and dirty? You let me go through a lot of trouble to fix my teeth, to get my hair cut, buy new clothes and get married." There was a long silence and then God spoke, "Morris, you look so much improved, I didn't recognize you!"

MY BRAIN

Since the day I started taking Lipitor I have noticed that it affected my brain. What I mean is that sometimes I don't remember names that I used to know. This was like having a hole in my memory. I could see the person's face or know his character, but I could not recall his name.

Last night I woke up at 2:00 AM to go to the bathroom. When I returned to bed I could not go to sleep. I tried several methods to induce sleep, but no luck! Then I decided to make my brain tired to allow me to go sleep. I started by remembering the names of all the fifty states of the U.S.A.

When I got to New Hampshire I could not remember the name "*New Hampshire*". I knew this is a state north of Massachusetts and south of Maine. But it name would not come to me. I said to my brain, "Now it is 2:00 AM. Leave me alone! Why do you want to know this name at this time? What is the emergency?" But my brain was not accepting no for an answer. It insisted to know the name, right then and there. I did not know what to do.

Then I remembered that there was a solution. Ask Miss Siri. I got out of bed and in the dark tip-toed to my cell phone and I called Siri. At the same time, I was making sure that my wife would not wake up. I asked Siri my question. She started with a loud voice telling me, "Hmmm, I have to think about it." Then a few seconds later she gave me the answer.

But now I had a different problem, my wife had been awakened and wanted to know what is her name and why I was calling her at this time of night!

MY SOUL

I had a dream last night that I was dead. I was floating in a vast, dark space that had no beginning and no end. It was very dark. I could not see or hear anything. Suddenly I realized that I was lost. I said to myself, "What will happen to me if I cannot get back to earth? Do I have to stay floating in this purgatory forever? Besides no one would know where I am?" I got so frightened that I woke up in a cold sweat.

I think in that vast space I will be like a drop of rain accompanied with many other drops returning to our origin, the immense sea. There I will be a minuscule drop. I would not be able to find any of my beloved relatives and friends.

In that sea, all souls are swimming without their individual personality and without a traceable past. No one would know them. The only thing left of them in this earth would be their descendants who would remember them hopefully and pray for them.

NOBODY LISTENS TO ME

I have three children and five grandchildren. None of them listens to my advice. Of course, I want only good things for them and I wish to save them from all harm but they don't listen to me.

I have done a lot of living and have accumulated a lot of experience but they think I am from the old school and my advice is old like out of fashioned clothes.

One of my grandsons is twenty years old and a student at an Ivy League university. He decided in his junior year to go abroad study a semester and enjoy a new culture. I thought he would choose an old European school like the University of Paris, or London but he decided to go to Tanzania. I said to him, "Tanzania is not a Mecca of science. It is a place to go on safari to see savage animals or to buy precious colored stones like Tanzanite. I did advise against this idea but as usual, no one listened to me.

He went there anyway and on his first day, he got bitten by a dog that was suspected of having Rabies. Then he contracted malaria and later typhoid fever. Thank God he finished the semester and returned to the United States. But of course, he did not remember my advice.

His cousin, a nineteen-year-old girl, was studying psychology at Kings College in London, England. During her summer vacation, she decided to go to South Korea for a semester of study abroad. I said to her, "Don't you know there is a war going on there? Why there? Korea is not a Mecca of Advanced Psychology!" But as usual, no one listens to me.

Finally, I came to the conclusion, they don't think that my advice is worth anything and I better keep my ideas to myself. Let them make their own mistakes and learn, as I did when I was young!

ODOMETER

Each car has an odometer that measures the number of miles that car has been driven. The number of miles goes up and up until the odometer is full. Then someone has to come and change it – maybe back to zero or maybe to 20,000 miles. The human being also has an odometer that has a certain capacity. Eventually, it will get full and cannot go any farther.

I was thinking that someday someone may be able to decrease the human odometer and lower its level and then man can live his life over and over.

Then I started daydreaming about which level I would like my odometer decreased to. I did not want to start at zero and go through childhood again. I wanted to start at age twenty. Then I continued my daydreaming asking myself what I would do if I were that age again?

I thought instead of going to Paris, France to study medicine I would go to Stanford University in California where the weather is nicer. I would study philosophy and become a philosopher. I wouldn't have to get up every morning at 6:00 AM and be in the operating room working under those harsh, hot lights in a tense atmosphere. I would not have the responsibility of people's lives in my hands.

Instead, I will be the professor of philosophy. I will get up at 9:00 AM, go to the office, sip coffee all day talking to students and academicians. I will spend my life in a relaxed atmosphere. I would not be on call in the Emergency Room and carry a beeper at all times.

When my daydreaming finished I felt this type of life might not be a happy one for me. This will not be a life of service to others. It would be a life without challenge and excitement.

Then I decided that I don't want anybody to change my odometer. If I have to live my life over again, I will do exactly what I have done in the past and with no regrets.

OPEN MOUTH PHENOMENON

I don't know why old people's mouths are always open. It doesn't matter if they are walking or sitting or lying down, or even listening to music.

I have several theories:

1. That old people are retired and sit around and talk constantly. Therefore they get tired, then when they rest their mouth stays open.
2. They are victims of chronic fatigue syndrome. When their bodies rest, their mouths lose the power of contraction and remain open.
3. When people get old, their nose gets blocked, therefore they have to keep their mouths open to breathe.
4. Maybe the time has changed so much, and they are so astonished by this evolution that their mouths are opened to show their astonishment.
5. Maybe no one listens to old people and they are continuously asking,

"Why?", "Why?"

PERFECTION

Many of the over eighties believe that since they have lived so long they deserve to have a perfect life to the end. They demand perfection. Especially if they have some savings.

Starting from their brain, they want a perfect memory. In order to achieve this, they buy many expensive over-the-counter medications and put themselves through a lot of pain trying to solve difficult puzzles.

Next they think about their eyes. They want their cataracts to be done by a famous ophthalmologist, using special lens costing over $6,000 dollars extra.

They want the latest hearing aids, the ones that transform sound to light and then light to sound. These cost much more than routine hearing aids.

They want their heart to work like when they were a teenager. So they want the latest aortic and mitral valves to be inserted in their heart.

They cannot tolerate any back pain so they want the latest minimally invasive back operations that cost a lot. They have no tolerance for any discomfort and pain.

The question is how the over eighties of twenty years

ago dealt with these problems, since none of these modern medical technologies were available.

The human body is like an old car. You can only do so much. The owner should be satisfied if it moves. I believe all the over eighties should be happy and satisfied that they are alive.

They can talk and walk and move like an old car. They will never be perfect like when they were young!

PLEADING

Naples, Florida has more old people than anywhere in the world.... or at least this is my opinion. The service industry is thriving. But getting actual service is another thing. When I moved to my new apartment I needed Comcast to fix my telephone, television, and internet. I called them but my telephone call did not do any good because it went to an answering machine. After waiting for two days and not receiving any response I had to call two more times to get a living soul. Is it normal to call at least two or three times to solve a problem?

Finally, when I got a live person on the line I explained my problem. She said the first appointment is in four weeks. Then I started to plead – like asking God for a favor! This did not do any good. I mentioned my age and my disability but this didn't do any good either. Finally it was a victory that at least I get an appointment in three weeks instead of four weeks!

One week before the appointment I received a call from a man with a severe Indian accent. He asked me if I still wanted the service or if my problem had been resolved. I asked if he was calling me from India. He said, "No, I am calling from

Philadelphia." I mentioned that he had an Indian accent and he replied that he was originally from Mexico. I said to him, "Whatever you do, please don't cancel my appointment, otherwise I will develop a nervous breakdown and you will be responsible for paying all my psychiatric bills."

Then I started counting the days until the appointment date. An operator called from Florida. She said the technician will be in your apartment sometime today between 2 to 6 p.m. I started pleading again that in that four-hour window I will be a prisoner in my house but this didn't do any good either.

At 5 p.m. the technician arrived. He was tired and cranky. This was his last call. But when he started to work I finally felt that I had won the battle. When I was young these things did not bother me. Now as an old man, it is unbearable!

PREDICTION

Fifty years ago no one in the world could tell a pregnant lady whether her child was going to be a boy or a girl. But since that time science has progressed and thanks to the art of Sonography now with almost certainty an expert can predict the sex of the baby.

With this story in mind, I said to myself that maybe fifty years from now with the help of supercomputers and medical past and family history, an expert could predict with reasonable certainty the exact date of death.

Continuing to dream farther I said, "If I know the exact date of my death, what would I do?" The first thing I would do: one day before the appointed date, I will give a very large dinner party and ask all of my friends to eulogize me. I want to enjoy hearing all the good things they would say. I am sure that since I am sitting in the audience they are not going to say anything bad.

The second thing I would do: two months before my death, I would start gradually giving away my wealth to charity. I don't want to give everything away at once because if there is an error in the date of my death then I will be destitute.

The last thing I will do: on the day of my death I will give everything away.

Some people may decide to commit some unusual act if they know this is the last day of their life. For example, one of my surgical colleagues was unreasonably sued. He was not upset with the patient, but he was angry at his lawyer. He told me, "If I know I have incurable cancer and my death is imminent, I will go to that S.O.B. lawyer's office and will punch him in the face to maim him forever.

I stopped dreaming and I came back to my skin. I said, "Thank God science has not gone that far yet and I don't have to make any decisions!

RETIREMENT

I hated the word "Retirement". I felt that only sissies retired. The weak people retired. The real man doesn't retire. He works until he drops. I thought that retirement was a cop-out. But then things changed.

Due to restrictions by managed care and other health insurance companies, regulations by the state and federal governments, and fear of malpractice, I came to the conclusion that the time was right to swallow my pride and retire.

But in reality, I did not want to retire. I loved my work and I loved my patients and in return, they loved me back. I wrote a letter to all of them that the time had come for me to retire and they should come to my office during the week of September 20th to receive their medical records. I did not want to sell my practice and receive complaints from patients that my replacement doctor did not treat them right.

The week of goodbye came. The atmosphere was happy and sad. It was a combination of a birthday party and a funeral. My patients were happy for me and at the same time crying when they were saying goodbye.

Now almost a decade later I still miss my previous work. I dream often that I am operating but when I wake up I am happy I don't have that responsibility! Even today when I hear about upcoming medical news I am glued to the TV and wanting to understand and observe whatever is there. Sometimes I feel jealous that I am not involved in the care of patients as other doctors are. At the end of the day I realize that I did not save any lives. I did not encourage and console any patients. I did not give any good news to the family. The only thing I did was to take care of myself. Then I regret it a lot.

But I console myself by saying, "You have done your work for thirty-nine years. You have accomplished your goals. Now is the time for the new generation of doctors to do their things. The torch has been passed to *The New Generation*!"

SEX AND OVER EIGHTIES

"Horny old broad and dirty old man" is out and sex for the aged is in. No longer is this subject taboo.

Adult children of the older parent think that it is gross! If this is good for them, why not for the parents.

According to the Bureau of Statistics in the U.S.A. in the year 2000, for every one person over the age of sixty-five, there were ten young adults. But in the year 2030, for every one person over sixty-five, there will be only five young adults.

As you see the number of the elderly is increasing every day. Their needs will change and society will have to accept the changing ideas about sex.

Sexuality is set at an early age and stays with us forever. The removal of sex organs such as the ovaries or testicles during adult life does not change the desire for sexual activities. Or if these organs are old and poorly functioning, still the desire may continue.

Testosterone is back again in the ordinary man's jargon. Everywhere on television, radio, and newspapers, there are advertisements about it and its effects. Low testosterone is common among older men. Some members of the *Geriatric*

Tribe get testosterone injections every month. They claim it makes them sexually active.

One of the over eighties from Long Island told me, "My doctor injects me with testosterone every month and the result is wonderful! It makes me chase my wife all around the house.

I talked to him about the dangers of this medication - such as stroke, cancer of the prostate and breast.

But his response was that "It's better to enjoy today, and not worry about tomorrow!"

SEXUAL HARASSMENT

I understand the meaning of "Sexual Harassment" but I don't know at what point it starts to be that. What is the minimum and what is the maximum harassment?

If a man sees a female colleague in the office corridor and he tells her, "I like the color of your lipstick and you look nice in your yellow blouse" – is this sexual harassment?

The definition of sexual harassment has changed in the last thirty years. I remember in the operating room, the surgeon would joke with the nurses and they would like it and even they would participate in the jokes. But if we did that today, it would be a "No, No" and we would be accused of sexual harassment.

Because of the recent increase in cases of sexual harassment many executives don't want to meet with young female employees in their offices and are now forced to meet them in some public place like a coffee shop. This backlash makes them think twice about whether or not to employ females.

I remember when I was practicing as a breast surgeon. I used to examine my patients alone without the presence of a nurse. Then because of so many accusations against physicians, I was forced to hire a female nurse to accompany me in the examining room. I was quite uncomfortable because in my opinion and my upbringing the examining room was sacred and it was a temple of trust.

One day when I went to the examining room accompanied by my nurse, a patient who I had known for some time told me, "Doctor, does she have to be here?" I said to myself, "Yes, she has to be here to tame me so I don't attack you like a savage animal or at the minimum I don't lick you like a cat." But of course, I didn't tell her what I was thinking. I said, "Yes, she has to be here. This is a new rule."

The meaning of sexual harassment is different in each country. In France, they would take it as a compliment, not an insult. In Paris when a woman went to the gynecologist there were not so many sheets to cover her during the examination.

But when I came to the U.S. the first time, as an intern, I went to examine a female, the nurse covered her with so many sheets that I could not find the organ that I wanted to examine. Now I see the difference from one country to another.

Vive la France.

SILVER PILLS

In Iran and in most Middle Eastern countries, a light complexion is very much in demand. Girls with a whiter complexion will have more suitors! In Persian, they say she is *Sefid Bolouri*. It means "crystal white".

My mother already had five children when at the age of thirty-one she became pregnant with me. She wanted very much that her baby will be born with a very white complexion. My grandfather, who lived with my parents found out about it and decided to help.

One day he went to the Bazar to consult with the drug maker to find a solution for his daughter-in-law. This man who had a lot of experience in herbal medicine told my grandfather, "The lady should take silver pills." Then he proceeded to grind a piece of silver and made ninety pills. Then he said, "She should take one pill a day for ninety days." My mother, of course, did not question her father-in-law and everyday swallowed a pill for three months. When I was born, I was not as white as they hoped but I was lighter than my brother.

Now eighty-seven years later, among all my siblings I am the one who has lived longer and I have had fewer health problems. My theory is that the silver pills did it! None of my sisters and brother received the same pills. Silver given to pregnant women during her first trimester does it make her children live longer?

There has been no double-blind study done on this subject by researchers but this theory sounds good to me!

SLEEP

Every night I go to bed about 9:30 PM and fall asleep immediately. I don't use any sleeping pills nor even a tylenol.

I am a good sleeper. I can sleep in the car, on the plane, at the hotel. The only place I cannot sleep is when I am swimming.

Interest in sleep changes with age. Children never want to go to sleep and young people are the same. Middle-aged people are very much interested in sleeping but they don't want to admit it because they will be labeled as old.

For a very long time the feeling of the medical community was that the elderly cannot sleep well because of psychological issues. Recently a study conducted by physicians of Beth Israel Deconess Hospital in Boston showed the real reason: there is a group of specific clusters of neurons in the brain that are associated with center of sleep. They slowly dying off as we get older.

This really is not good news because getting sleep will get harder and harder as we age. So far there is no medication to regenerate this group of neurons in the brain.

The over eighties compensate by taking naps during the day. I personally have been taking naps every afternoon for many years, even when I was working as a surgeon. a little nap and a cup of tea did a lot of good.

Tossing and turning in bed at night is not a good idea. Instead getting up and doing something productive is much better. This way one can accomplish a task and then this will help him to sleep easier later on.

When I sleep I dream constantly. My life during the dream is very colorful and exciting, however my life when I am awake is routine and calm. I am fortunate to live two lives. During the waking time I am Dr. Jekyll and at night I am Mr. Hyde. In the morning I am so exhausted from all my adventures that I have to recover from my escapades gradually.

My wife said I talk in my sleep but she doesn't know whether it is in English, Persian or French. The only thing she knows is that she doesn't understand a word. She hopes that it is not about her.

SNEEZE

I was taking a plane from St. Louis, MO. to San Francisco, CA. I had made the reservation on Southwest Airlines that does not have first class seats. All seats are grouped three on each side of the aisle. When my wife and I entered the plane, we looked for seats. We found that row 12 had two empty seats, one by the window and the other in the middle.

A woman about 60 was already sitting on the aisle. She was wearing a two pieced dark blue suit. Her bright red lipstick was an indication of her wanting to be younger than she was. Her salt and pepper hair was pulled back in a chignon. She had a pair of heavy rim glasses and a bright red U-shaped pillow around her neck to make her more comfortable when she fell asleep.

She stood up and reluctantly let us pass to our seats. I took another look at her to get a second opinion. I found her looking very prim and proper, almost like an old Smith College graduate. However, she did not pay any attention to me. There was no glance, no smile and no hello. She continued reading her book as if we did not exist.

After the plane took off and about one hour in the air, I started to sneeze. My sneezes are usually loud. I have no control over them. They come one after the other like a machine gun, at the least five to seven times. Sometimes they come in intervals of one to two minutes.

After my first sneeze, I saw in her face a sign of discomfort. When one minute later the second one arrived, she pulled away to the edge of her seat. I was sure she was telling herself, this guy has a cold and I am going to catch it. When the third one arrived, she appeared aggravated. She reached for her purse that was under the seat, opened the zipper and pulled out a hand activated nebulizer. She took two puffs of it.

Everything was calm for the next few minutes when suddenly the fourth sneeze came. I looked at her again and she had such a sour face that I did not have the audacity to tell her, "Lady, I am not sick, but be prepared, my routine is five to seven sneezes so still expect three more to com!"

When the fifth one arrived she looked at me for the first time. I'm sure she saw my dark complexion and she must have told herself, "Now I am in real trouble. He must be from Africa and he could possibly have Ebola virus." However, at this point, there was nothing she could do. The plane was packed and there wasn't a possibility of changing seats.

In desperation again, she opened her purse and pulled out her very bright lipstick and refreshed her lips. I supposed she was hoping that it had some antiviral material in it that would kill the Ebola virus. Fortunately for her, I stopped sneeze at number five. Then she relaxed, put back her seat and with her red pillow around her neck, fell asleep.

STOCKS

Playing stocks for the over eighties is a very dangerous game. Everybody will tell you that it is like gambling. Also, they tell you that when you play this game, you should only play with the money that you don't need.

I don't know how many times I have entered the stock market and lost money. But then restarted a few years later! I buy stocks and the value goes down. Even if the price was already a bargain, I sell the stock and immediately the price goes up!

Even a donkey knows better. When he walks and falls in the hole, next time, he does not repeat the same mistake and goes around the hole. But the human with two legs cannot learn the lesson.

The reason is friends and the media – especially – *"Mad Money"* on television. He encourages people to buy. He says good things regarding a special stock. Then the next day the price goes up because everyone blindly follows his advice. Then two days later the price goes down.

The market is manipulated by the big boys. We the little people, the over eighties, have no chance.

In spite of it all, occasionally I get encouraged to buy stocks, knowing that for sure the value will go down.

I guess I have not learned from the donkey's experience. There is no hope!

STUBBORNNESS

Over eighties generally are stubborn but they don't call it stubbornness. They call it *"perseverance"*. There is a great difference between the two. The dictionary definition of stubbornness is: "Show dogged determination; not to change one's attitude or position in spite of good argument or reason to do so." The definition of perseverance is: "steadfastness in doing something despite difficulty in achieving success."

I wanted to write a story regarding this subject to clarify what stubbornness really means. Recently I was talking about it to a friend. She said, "My husband and I while traveling alternate and share the driving. One early morning I was the driver. My husband continuously commented on my driving: "You are going to fast! Watch out for police. Watch for crossing animals. There are wild animals in this region that may jump out in front of our car."

I was getting irritated. I said, "Each time you make a comment, I will accelerate ten more miles." This continued up until I was going over 100. He said, "I don't want to be killed on this strange road. Stop the car! I want to get out." I suddenly brought the car to a stop and opened the passenger side door for him to exit." Yes, this was a true example of cutting off your nose to spite your face. Indeed, it was stupid stubbornness.

What is the remedy for this disease? I believe an open discussion and consultation as has been recommended and practiced in the Baha'i Faith.

SURGICAL OPERATION

The old person's body is like an old building. It foundation is cracked and the bricks are loose. If someone pulled out a few of these bricks it's possible that the whole building would fall.

A surgical operation for over eighties is dangerous. It certainly is a shock to the body, and is stressful. General anesthesia has its own complications, both physically and mentally.

If you put all of this together it will be similar to pulling out a few bricks from an old building. The outcome is grim.

I am a surgeon and naturally, I was trained to cut and operate but I do not advise any non-emergency elective operations for this group and certainly not any orthopedic procedure.

The reason is that we are dealing with a process of degenerative disease. If one part of the body is fixed it will be temporary. The condition of degeneration will continue forever. The same problem will come back. Maybe not in the same location, but close to it.

I have operated on many geriatric patients. People over ninety years of age do not tolerate surgical procedures. They may do well for one to three post-op days but then they run out of gas and die.

TELEPHONE

The telephone could be a friend when a loved one calls or it could be an enemy when an advertiser calls. These telemarketers are a nuisance. They intrude in your life at the most inopportune time and you cannot get rid of them. I have tried to block them, put them on the "do not call list", etc. But they always find a way to call me.

They especially like the over eighties because they know they have a lot of time and are the ideal victims. They call claiming they are from Microsoft and your computer needs a change in software. If you don't do it immediately the computer will freeze. I fell for it once and it caused a lot of problems for me.

Sometimes they call and say that they are an agent of the I.R.S. and you have to send a money order immediately.

Last year I received a call from a young man pretending to be my grandson. With a crying voice, he said, "Grandpa, I am in jail and they want $2,000 dollars to release me. Please, please help me!" I knew it was a fake. Why would he call me instead of his parents? I said to him, "I hope they will keep you in jail forever!"

I call my children on and off. Some of them won't pick

up the phone at all even if they are standing next to it. They believe that the telephone is an enemy. Usually, I leave a detailed message and ask to be called back immediately. They call two days later. I asked them, "Did you listen to my message?" They tell me, "No, I just saw your telephone number and I called." I said, "I wasted my time and energy leaving a complete message!"

This is the way the next generation lives. Now if they don't answer, I just hang up. I thought the remedy would be a text message and it would attract their attention but it did not work all the time.

THE CHOSEN PEOPLE

Over eighties are the chosen people. In the United States, thirty percent of people aged twenty do not make it to the age of eighty. Only 3.4 percent of the world's population is over the age of eighty.

This group of over eighties is a very special select group. Indeed they are the chosen people. Most of them have been through a lot of pain and jumped through a lot of hoops to get to the age of eighty.

Starting from birth, a certain number died at delivery; one to two percent died in infancy; five percent died of childhood diseases. In adolescence, another five percent do not make it. Then between thirty to sixty years, another ten percent die of heart, cancer, stroke, infectious diseases. From age sixty to eighty, eleven percent more die. This makes a total of twenty-eight percent. Therefore, only seventy-two percent make it to the age of eighty.

Indeed, they are the chosen people and must be respected as the Veterans of the "War of Life". They did not come back from killing fields but they returned from the battle of life with mental and physical scars forever.

They should be honored!

THE DENTIST

I was sent by my dentist to see the oral surgeon. I was given a note to be delivered to him. It said, "Cut his bridge located in the upper jaw and remove his number 15 tooth."

When I entered his office, the waiting room was like a room in the Palais de Versailles. It was decorated with furniture of Louis de 15th epoch. I said to myself, "For sure his fee will be high!" As I sat, I started to look around. Then I saw his name in large letters in his diploma on the wall. At this time I became very frightened because he was the same surgeon who extracted the wrong tooth of one of my friends. Now I was going to have the same procedure done! Could the same thing happen to me?

I was fidgeting in my chair when they called me to the consultation room. The place was also tastefully decorated with colorful curtains and a lot of modern painting on the wall. After a few minutes, the surgeon walked in. He was tall and very muscular, looked more like a football player. After he examined me, I told him that I didn't want sedation, only local anesthesia, because I wanted to make sure he didn't remove the wrong tooth.

The day of surgery, I got up early in the morning. As soon

as I arrived to the office the secretary handed me two pages of consent forms. In the forms, they talked about paralysis of the face, lacerations of mouth and tongue and nerve injury. I was okay with all of this. Then I got to the section regarding pregnancy. I told the secretary that this did not apply to me. She said, "You have to initial everything it doesn't matter what. These are my orders. If any of them are left blank you won't be having the operation today. I signed them all, including to promise to stop my birth control pills and notify my doctor if I don't.

Finally, I was ready. The surgeon did what he was supposed to do under my suspicious eyes. He did not remove the wrong tooth. When I was done, they took me back to the same secretary and she presented me with the bill which is what the French call "*La Dolourose,*" - *The Painful.*

Indeed it was quite high and had to be paid immediately!

THE ELEVATOR

My son who lives in New York was celebrating the Birth of Bahá'u'lláh by having a party in his house. He had invited 75 people: old, young, white and black, and from many different nationalities.

I was standing at the front door welcoming many of my old friends, most of whom I had not seen for some time. Among them was an older woman about 65. She was elegantly dressed in a two piece light blue colored suit. Her hair was cut short which made her look younger. She shook hands with me.

Then she said, "Do you know who I am?" I looked at her for a second time but I could not recognize her. Then she said, "I am Linda, an old friend and one of your former patients." Then suddenly like a bolt of lightning striking me I remembered her. I said, "What happened to you? You've lost a lot of weight?" She replied, "One year ago I had gastric bypass surgery and it transformed me. I lost 170 pounds! As the result, I no longer need to take any medication."

After a short conversation, she left to join the other guests. I tried to reminisce and remember the Dorothy who I knew long ago. She was very overweight, puffy face and chronically tired. Now she was transformed into a beautiful, mature and alive woman. Thinking of Dorothy made me remember the story of 'The Elevator'.

One day Jacob and his 12-year-old son from the Pennsylvania Dutch Country decided to visit Philadelphia. They had never been in a big city. They went to Bloomingdale's Department store. Everything they saw was a novelty for them. They saw An elderly, overweight woman bent over and walking with a cane entered a box located in the middle of the store. This was the (elevator cab). The box door closed behind her. They continued looking at the box not knowing what happened to the old woman.

Then after five minutes the door of the box opened and a very beautiful young lady with flowing blond hair and walking very straight, without a cane, came out. Father and son were fascinated by this transformation. Then the father said to his son, "Run and get your mother and bring her here. She must go into this box!"

THE SWIMMER

In the middle of May when the weather was hot, I decided to go swimming in the sea in front of our apartment building. It was about 3 p.m. when I got to the sidewalk. Before descending the stairs to the beach I noticed in the distance a blond was swimming going away from the beach. She had long, blond platinum hair that with each wave, floated side to side. I had never seen any woman swim so fast.

I was fascinated by her powerful stroke and fast speed. Yet I was worried that she may be going too far out and get into trouble. Then suddenly, like someone had sent her an urgent message, she turned around and started to swim back towards the shore.

As she got closer, she stood up. Now the water was at the level of her shoulders. Since the water was very clear and transparent I could see her entire body clearly. I was surprised to see that she was not wearing any top. Her breasts were of an adequate size, perky and not droopy. As a breast specialist, I wanted clinically to evaluate them by inspection. I thought if anyone would do the "Pencil Test" it would most certainly be positive and the pencil would fall into the water.

I said to myself, does she not know that this isn't a Nudist

Colony or a topless beach? Then I remembered that when I was in St. Tropez in the south of France, many girls did not wear a top. But Naples is a very conservative town and it is not the French Riviera. I thought that at any moment the police will come and arrest her but no such luck.

As she started to walk towards me and I was standing at the edge of the water, I could see not only her long blond hair, but also I could see a lot of hair on her chest. At this point, I decided to look again and maybe get a second opinion. But there was no need for that when I saw his tiny bikini.

Now, I was downright angry at him. I wasted my time. There was no way I could get back my enjoyable fantasy and admiration. I wanted to tell him that he shouldn't cheat people like this. He should either shave his head and get rid of that gorgeous hair or he should have a bilateral mastectomy.

But I did not tell him any of this. Instead, I plunged myself into the sea and tried to cool off my anger.

THE TICKET

I am not computer literate. In fact, until two years ago I was not able to use a computer at all. I was really afraid of them. But necessity forced me to learn. I said to myself, "I should move up to the 21st Century." And no excuses.

Then I started to type, but not like everyone else. I type with my index finger, one word at a time. Good thing my grandchildren could not see me.

This morning I decided to get our airline tickets to go to Minnesota. I got on the phone and called American Airlines. After ten minutes of listening to their music, finally, a woman answered. I said, "I want to get two round-trip tickets to Minnesota and I want to use my miles to pay for them."

After everything was set she said, "There is a twenty-five dollar charge for each ticket if it is done by me." Then she said, "Why don't you go on the internet and save yourself fifty dollars." I said, "How difficult is it?" She said, "Nothing to it. The computer will direct you." I hung up with her.

With great enthusiasm, I got on the internet and started answering all the questions for my booking. I was feeling lucky until I got to the question asking for my password. Of course, I didn't know it. I spent so much time trying to find my password that my time ran out and I had to start all over again. Finally, with a lot of painful moments spent in front of the computer I finished. The end result: The computer said your ticket would cost $550.00. I said, "No, no! I want to use my miles."

In desperation, I called back American Airlines and after waiting again for 17 minutes a woman told me that she could not help me. If you want to use your miles, I can do it for you for $25.00 each ticket. Otherwise, you have to redo all your information. At this point, I was exhausted. I could not tolerate having to redo my itinerary. I said to the woman, "I will pay, please do it for me".

When everything was finished I remembered a Persian story that fits my situation.....

"A man has committed a crime and he was brought before the judge. The judge said for the punishment I give you three choices: 1) You can receive 100 lashes, 2) You can eat five pounds of onions, 3) Pay $500.00 fine. The man said, "I think I can tolerate 100 lashes." They started to administer the lashes. After ten lashes he couldn't take anymore. He said, "Stop! I will eat the raw onion." Then after eating four onions, he couldn't eat another one. Then he said, "I will pay the $500.00."

In my case, I should have paid the $50.00 at the beginning and not have gone through all the stressful moments in front of the computer!

THERMOMETER

A few days ago, I started to have a runny nose and a scratchy throat. I could not believe that in Florida I would catch a cold because I came to this sunny state to be immune from this kind of illness. The next day I felt hot. I asked my wife to check my forehead to see if I had a fever. She did it a few times. Sometimes she said yes, you have a fever, sometimes she said maybe, and sometimes she said not at all. Finally, she got sick and tired of using her clinical judgement by this crude method and wanted to know why as an educated man – a physician – I wasn't using a thermometer?

I looked all over my apartment and couldn't find one. As I felt really crummy and didn't want to go to the drug store I called Gita and asked her to buy me one. I told her I wanted something very simple, like the ones we used in Iran.

But the thermometer that Gita bought was very different from the Middle Ages ones we used to own. This one was wrapped up in a thick plastic cover and on it was written: "Fast Reading Digital Clinical Thermometer". I looked at it again, it was packaged like a very high-tech item. I tried to open it but I couldn't do it because it was very tightly sealed. Maybe the manufacturers thought someone might try to put some kind of poison into the package and the user would die before he could ever know his temperature!

I went to the kitchen and got a razor and a knife and finally with great difficulty opened the package and got the thermometer out. I said to my wife, "I was looking for a simple thermometer like the one that I had been using for the past 50 years, the one that you shake hard until the mercury drops below 86 degrees Fahrenheit. You put it under your tongue, wait about five minutes and then look at it in many different directions to see the level of the mercury. If you have good eyesight you probably would be able to read your body temperature."

But the one that I got was not the same. It had a four-page booklet of instructions on how to use it. As usual, I didn't read any of it. I put the thermometer under my tongue and after a few minutes, I looked to see the result. It didn't show anything. At this point, I had no choice. I had to read the instructions all the while protesting as to why I should be forced to do so.

The instructions read, first you have to activate the instrument, when it showed the number eight four times, put it in your mouth. There was a diagram showing exactly where in your mouth you should put it. Then press the button and wait for 25 seconds. The display window will change color several times and finally, your temperature will appear. But, you have to hurry to read it. If you don't have your reading glasses with you, the number will disappear, and you have to start all over again. I said to myself, I don't want this high tech instrument that you have to have a Ph.D. in engineering to understand it. I want my old mercury probe that I used for so many years. Unfortunately, they don't make those anymore. You can't find them and they are considered an antique.

TIN CUP

One of the major preoccupations of the elderly is their financial situation. They want to know if they are going to have enough money to live on until the end of their life. In my case, thank God, I have enough money. But there is a technical problem.

According to the Federal Government's Actuarial calculation, I have to take money out of my retirement plan every year. This way gradually my retirement money will decrease. By the time I get to be 100 years old, there will be no more money left in my retirement plan.

In the same situation, I have sold a piece of real estate some time ago and every month I get a fixed sum of money until I am 100 years old. At that age, there will be no money left in the account.

Also, I am receiving a social security check every month. I am not sure if when I get to be 100 there will be any money left in the Treasury. What should I do when I am 100 and one days old? I have given this situation a lot of thought. I came to a very interesting solution.

When I get to the age of 100 and no more money will

come to me routinely, with my small reserve I will buy a tin cup. Then I will go and sit in front of the Silver Spot movie house and ask people to drop some change in my cup. But hopefully, this will never happen!

VISION

Seeing is a God-given right. Everybody wants to see good, especially over eighties. Reading is one of the pleasures of their lives. They want to have 20/20 vision and nothing less! For this reason, they will go through any operation - the fanciest, the most expensive with the latest technology. They are willing to travel to the end of the world to find the specialist of their choice.

One of my friends needed a cataract operation. The first thing he did was to get the name of all ophthalmologists in Naples. Then he went to the internet and researched their education, what medical school they graduated from and where they had their residency and fellowship training. After this extensive evaluation, he chose one.

The doctor told him, "I can do the regular cataract operation and have Medicare pay for it 100 percent. But if you want me to use my latest machinery and latest cutting-edge technology this will cost $3000 dollars more." Of course, my friend chose the latter.

After the fancy operation was done by the doctor who was a Harvard graduate, my friend could only see double and not as good as pre-operatively. He went back and forth to the doctor but there was no improvement.

The upshot was that the ophthalmologist got frightened that he might be sued so he sent a letter to my friend telling him that he no longer wanted him as a patient and he recommended the name of another ophthalmologist.

This tells us that you should not expect 100 percent good results at this age. The risk goes up with age. Sometimes it's better to be satisfied with what you already have.

Another case is of my accountant. He could not taste his food well because of nasal polyps. He went to the best specialist in New York City. After the operation, he found that the surgeon had injured the nerve going to his eye. He lost the use of one eye and his taste did not improve either.

At the age of over eighty, do not look for perfection!

WHO IS AN OLD MAN?

I was seriously searching to find out who should be called old? What is the qualification of someone that we call old? I looked for the answer in the dictionary. It said, "The old person is someone who is no longer young and has lived for a long time." But this did not satisfy me.

Then I talked to my friends. One of them said, "Old is someone who is fifteen years older than you are." I liked his definition. But still, this was not what I was looking for. Then I asked my imagination who is an old man?

This was the response: "He is bald, with a few white hairs for sideburns. His face has a lot of wrinkles. His neck has extra skin like a turkey's neck. His chest is like a barrel and his abdomen protrudes like a drum. His rectal sphincter is incompetent. He walks bent over with a cane."

I did not like him at all and I felt it was my duty to change him! But how? Then I remembered how I advised the old Scottish man when I recently was in Edinburgh, Scotland.

There I went to a variety show and one of the songs was about a son singing to his father. At the same time, they were projecting the image of his father who was looking sad and exhausted.

He was wearing a long, turned up coat and he was sitting on a bench in the street like a homeless man. When I saw him I said to myself, "It is entirely the old man's fault, to think he is old and to dress in shabby clothing. He should snap out of it, change his appearance and think that he is young. He certainly doesn't need his son's pity and singing!"

Then I came to the conclusion that the old man should continuously fight against the feeling that he is old. He should not accept it. He should keep his mind and body active and certainly keep his appearance as excellent as possible!

YOUNG AGAINST OLD

Every afternoon when I watch T.V. whether it's CNBC or CNN I am interrupted by their advertisements. Most of the time they are stupid ads beneath the dignity of human beings. The only rewarding part is seeing the young girls who participate in these advertisements.

They are all the same type. Mostly white with long blond hair, blue eyes and perfect body shapes. Occasionally, you see a Black or Latin girl. You never see an ugly or a fat girl and of course never an old lady.

These advertisements are directed mostly towards the people between the ages of eighteen to thirty-five. They don't direct them towards over eighties. They are ignoring them. They don't want to play with the oldies.

When I watch CNN I see the anchor girls and reporters are mostly young women. I never see old ladies with white hair and dull appearances. I am always impressed by the amount of knowledge these young women have. They are sharp when questioning old guys. There is no comparison between the young and old.

Today the world is run by the young people. They are in power. But don't worry, their time will come. They will get old, fat and ugly. Many years later when they announce their death they won't show their current picture, instead they show their picture when they were young. This is cheating.

Forget the racial battle between black and white. Now there is a battle between young and old. But according to the law of nature, the young will win.

They are the New Generation!

ABOUT THE AUTHOR

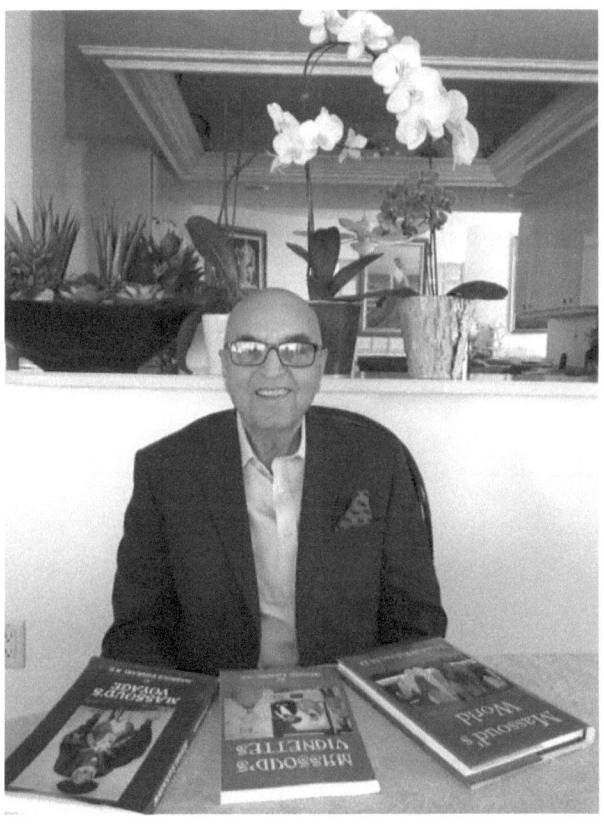

Dr. Massoud Eghrari was born in Tehran, Iran. He had his elementary and secondary school in that city. He graduated from the American High School of Tehran (Alborz). Supported by his parents, Haj Shaban and Baheyeh Khanun, he was sent to Paris, France to study medicine. He graduated from the University of Paris Medical School. He came to the United States to pursue his specialty in the field of surgery. He started his private practice of surgery in Smithtown, New York where he practiced for 39 years.

During this time, he became assistant professor of surgery at Stony Brook Medical School, President and then governor of the American College of Surgeons, Eastern Long Island Chapter.

His first marriage was to the late Isabella Belyea Ryan with whom he had three children Mark Shaban, Jacqueline Shirine and Carolyn Kian and five grandchildren. Dr. Eghrari now resides in Naples with his present wife Tayebeh (Manijeh).

He spends most of his time writing, painting and playing the santour (Persian musical instrument).

OTHER BOOKS PUBLISHED
BY THE AUTHOR

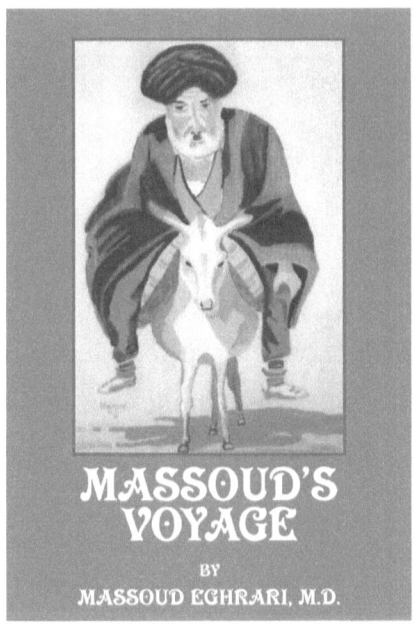

This is the second volume of Massoud's stories. This book contains seventy-five true short stories which take the reader through his slow, colorful travels from childhood to retirement, and reveal his philosophy of life. As the author's painting on the front cover illustrates, he likens his life's adventurous journey to a long, slow donkey ride over sometimes rough and rutted paths.

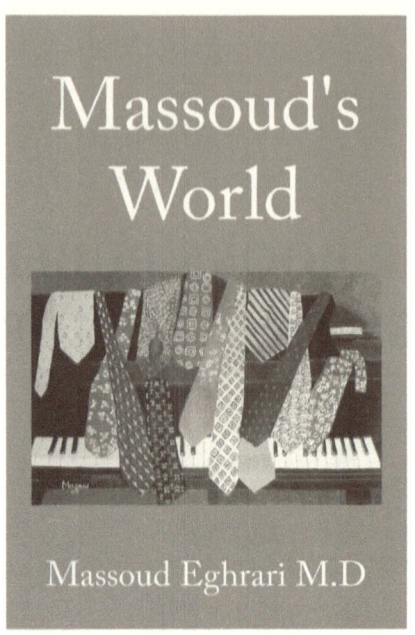

Massoud's World

Massoud Eghrari M.D

This is the third volume of Massoud's stories. This book contains seventy-nine short stories of his life experiences. As the Author's paintings on the front cover illustrates, he likens his stories to different shapes and colorful ties that he has worn during his professional life.

www.ingramcontent.com/pod-product-compliance
Lightning Source LLC
Chambersburg PA
CBHW020538290526
45786CB00002B/936